Cristiele Fiuza Soares
Janice Luehring G
Mirian Maria Caetano

Atividade antibiofilme do oleo de palmarosa (Cymbopogon martini)

Cristiele Fiuza Soares
Janice Luehring G
Mirian Maria Caetano

Atividade antibiofilme do oleo de palmarosa (Cymbopogon martini)

ScienciaScripts

Imprint
Any brand names and product names mentioned in this book are subject to trademark, brand or patent protection and are trademarks or registered trademarks of their respective holders. The use of brand names, product names, common names, trade names, product descriptions etc. even without a particular marking in this work is in no way to be construed to mean that such names may be regarded as unrestricted in respect of trademark and brand protection legislation and could thus be used by anyone.

Cover image: www.ingimage.com

This book is a translation from the original published under ISBN 978-613-9-64718-7.

Publisher:
Sciencia Scripts
is a trademark of
Dodo Books Indian Ocean Ltd. and OmniScriptum S.R.L publishing group

120 High Road, East Finchley, London, N2 9ED, United Kingdom
Str. Armeneasca 28/1, office 1, Chisinau MD-2012, Republic of Moldova, Europe
Printed at: see last page
ISBN: 978-620-7-78131-7

SUMMARY

Due to the increase in hospital infections, the resistance of pathogenic microorganisms and the lack of drugs to combat and inhibit their growth, new alternatives have been sought to combat these resistant microorganisms. Urinary tract infections are among the four most common types of hospital-acquired infections, which have contributed to higher morbidity and mortality rates, higher hospital costs and longer lengths of stay. These include infections caused by Candida spp., which represent a growing threat to human health, causing nosocomial infections and candidemia, which can lead to the patient's death. Its ability to form biofilm on inert surfaces, such as urinary catheters, is responsible for its high pathogenicity, since its occurrence triggers resistance to antifungal drugs. Palmarosa (Cymbopogon martini) is a species of aromatic grass grown for the extraction of essential oil. Due to its high geraniol content, it has various therapeutic properties, including its efficacy against insects, antimicrobial, anti-infectious, anti-tumour and immunomodulatory activity. Therefore, the aim of this study was to verify the antibiofilm activity of palmarosa oil against Candida albicans in urinary tubes. Strains of C. albicans were used to form biofilms on the urinary tubes and then treatment was carried out with the oil diluted by macrodilution with the concentration determined by MIC. Biofilm quantification was carried out using the classic CFU/mL counting method. The results showed that the oil at a concentration of $110gg/mL^{-1}$ had a significant response against C. albicans strains, demonstrating that in small concentrations, there is a relevant antifungal action. In addition, the oil showed significant antibiofilm activity against the biofilm formed by the C. albicans inoculum. Thus, with the results obtained in this study of the antifungal and antibiofilm action of palmarosa oil, it has become a new means of combating these resistant microorganisms and reducing hospital infection rates.

Keywords: Biofilm, Candida albicans, hospital infection.

SUMMARY

CHAPTER 1

INTRODUCTION

Essential oils are the volatile elements contained in plant organs, which play a fundamental role in defence against microorganisms (SIQUI et al., 2000). Around 60 per cent of essential oils have antifungal activity and 35 per cent antibacterial activity (BHAVANANI; BALLOW, 2000). Due to the rate of increase in the resistance of pathogenic microorganisms in hospital environments and microbial resistance to the drugs available on the market, new therapeutic alternatives have been sought in order to combat these resistant microorganisms, such as the use of essential oils for therapeutic purposes (NOVAIS et al., 2003; ANTUNES et al., 2006; OLIVEIRA et al., 2006; OLIVEIRA et al., 2007).

Palmarosa (Cymbopogon martini) is a plant that belongs to the Poaceae family. Most of the species belonging to this genus have essential oils with aromatic characteristics and are of commercial and industrial importance in cosmetics, perfumes and pharmaceutical applications (LORENZI, 2002). It is a plant native to India and cultivated on a large scale, especially in tropical and subtropical regions. Its main constituent is geraniol, which has been reported to have high antimicrobial activity (PATTNAIK et al., 1997; VAN ZYL et al., 2006; DUARTE et al., 2007; JIROVETZ et al., 2007).

Palmarosa is a very aromatic species of grass grown for the extraction of essential oil. Because of its main constituent geraniol, it has different pharmacological properties, including its effectiveness against insects, its antifungal action, such as against Candida albicans, antimicrobial, anti-infectious, antitumour and immunomodulatory activity (SCHERER et al., 2009; ALMEIDA et al., 2011).

Technological advances related to invasive procedures for diagnosis and treatment, as well as the emergence of microorganisms that are multi-resistant to commercially available antimicrobials, have made hospital-acquired infections a major public health problem. The incidence of hospital-acquired infections caused by bacteria has been increasing over the last few decades and is one of the main causes of morbidity and mortality, causing an increase in hospitalisation time and high costs associated with the treatment of seriously ill patients (GUDLAUGSSON et al., 2003; HOTA, 2004; BATISTA; RODRIGUES, 2012).

Studies have shown that factors related to health-related infections (HAIs) are caused by the use of medical devices or surgical implants, such as urinary catheters, central venous catheters, among others, which are sources of microbial infections (AZEVEDO; CERCA, 2012; GUDLAUGSSON, 2003). It used to be believed that microbial growth was considered to be in suspension, that particulate material was in motion. However, recent research indicates that most microbial populations tend to form aggregates of various species, forming a microbial community called a biofilm (AZEVEDO; CERCA, 2012; MCDOUGALD et al., 2012). Biofilm is characterised by irreversible cells adhered to a substrate or to each other and embedded in a matrix made up of extracellular polysaccharides of their own production (DONLAN, COSTERTON, 2002).

Species of the genus Candida have been the most frequently isolated agents and account for around 80 per cent of hospital-acquired fungal infections. These microorganisms are considered to be the fourth leading cause of blood infections and can lead to death in around 25 to 38% of patients who develop candidemia (CHENG et al., 2005). These microorganisms may be mainly related to the formation of biofilms on medical devices such as catheters, prostheses and probes (SIMÕES, 2011; PERCIVAL et al., 2012). In addition, their ability to form biofilms on various surfaces and their resistance to antifungal drugs has increased interest in the search for new alternatives to control and inhibit these infections (JARVIS, 1995).

Palmarosa oil is therefore an interesting therapeutic strategy to combat the formation of Candida spp. biofilms in urinary catheters. In this way, this study aims to verify the degree of antibiofilm activity of palmarosa oil in promoting significant inhibition of the microorganism, with the aim of reducing hospital infection rates and mortality rates.

CHAPTER 2

OBJECTIVES

1.1   General Objective

To evaluate the antibiofilm activity of palmarosa oil in urinary tubes against Candida albicans strains.

1.2   Specific objectives

- Carry out gas chromatography of palmarosa oil to check its main constituents;
- Determine the minimum inhibitory concentration of pure palmarosa oil;
- Evaluate the growth of *Candida albicans* biofilm on urinary catheters;
- To evaluate the antibiofilm activity of palmarosa oil against *Candida albicans* strains.

CHAPTER 3

THEORETICAL FRAMEWORK

3.1 Hospital infection

Patients who are hospitalised in healthcare institutions are exposed to a range of pathogenic microorganisms, especially in the Intensive Care Unit (ICU), where the use of invasive procedures and broad-spectrum, potent antimicrobials are routine (MOURA et al., 2007).

According to the Ministry of Health (MoH), Ordinance No. 2616 of 12 May 1998 defines hospital-acquired infection (HI) as an infection acquired shortly after a patient is admitted to a hospital and which manifests itself during hospitalisation or after discharge, when it can be related to hospitalisation or hospital procedures (MINISTÉRIO DA SAÚDE, 1998).

The problem of HI in Brazil is growing every day, and it can be considered that the cost of treating patients with HI is three times higher than the cost of patients without infection. Even with the legislation in force in the country, HI rates remain high, at 15.5 per cent, corresponding to 1.18 episodes of infection per patient hospitalised with HI in Brazilian hospitals. Furthermore, the fact that public health institutions have the highest prevalence rate of HI in the country at 18.4% (PRADE, 1995) is considered more aggravating.

Identifying the prevalence rate of hospital-acquired infections depends on the use of epidemiological surveillance techniques, the criteria of intrinsic and extrinsic risk factors and diagnosis in a given unit over a given period of time (COUTO et al., 2003).

ICUs are of paramount importance for providing two main services for critically ill patients: life support in cases of severe organ failure and abundant monitoring to enable early identification and appropriate treatment of serious clinical complications. They establish highly complex levels of health care, proceeding effectively when there is instability of organs and functional systems with a risk of death (MARTINS, 2006).

In this way, patients in the Intensive Care Unit are at 5 to 10 times greater risk of contracting an infection than those in other hospitalisation units, as well as being more vulnerable to infection because they are frequently exposed to risk factors (COUTO et al., 2003).

The incidence rates of hospital-acquired infections for patients in the ICU can vary according to the type of population cared for and the unit, due to the severity of the underlying disease, the restriction of patients in bed, the concomitant use of sedatives and changes in levels of consciousness and the following invasive procedures of the respiratory tract, with the main risk factor being the use of mechanical ventilation related to the length of time it is used, also including contamination of the equipment and solutions used in ventilation therapy, among others (COUTO et al., 2003), Other factors that may be associated are the use of an orotracheal tube, the presence of a bladder catheter, stress ulcer prophylaxis, multiple traumas, the use of a nasogastric tube and the use of a mechanical ventilator (MARTINS, 2006). But according to epidemiological data, 35% to 45% of all cases of hospital-acquired infections are urinary tract infections, 80% of which are associated with the use of indwelling bladder catheters (the main vehicle of transmission) (GUIMARÃES; ROCCO, 2006).

3.2 Urinary tract infections

Hospital-acquired infections are a major problem that has caused harm to public health, both in Brazil and worldwide. It constitutes a risk to the health of hospital users who undergo therapeutic or diagnostic procedures (LACERDA, 2003). Before the 20th century, there were no reports of invasive infections by yeasts of the genus Candida, but only in recent decades have species of Candida albicans and non-albicans species become increasingly significant as a cause of infections (OLIVEIRA et al., 2001).

The change of yeast from a commensal to an important agent of infection has occurred in hospital environments as a result of medical progress, such as the emergence of invasive procedures, breaking down natural protective barriers, the limited use of broad-spectrum antibiotics and the efficiency of sustaining the lives of debilitated people who are vulnerable to opportunistic microorganisms (EDWARDS, 1991). Due to these circumstances, the increase in local alterations favours the colonisation and fungal infection of the urinary tract, usually caused by Candida species, and which may have renal complications, such as abscesses and fungal ball, as well as systemic complications (BRYAN et al., 1999; DUPONT, 1991).

Urinary tract infections (UTIs) are among the four most frequent types of hospital-acquired infections and are characterised by the invasion of microorganisms into any tissue of the urinary tract (STAMM, 1991). A study carried out in American hospitals between 1980-1990 showed that Candida was the sixth most frequent agent of infections, rising to fourth when it came to the most common microorganisms in intensive care units (JARVIS, 1995). This study showed that the incidence of fungemia increased from 0.1/1000 patients to 0.5/1000 patients, and that the occurrence of fungal infections of the urinary tract increased from 0.9/1000 patients to 2.0/1000 patients, most of which were caused by Candida species. This showed that the main site of infection for this yeast was the urinary tract, implicated in 46% of cases (JARVIS, 1995).

This is responsible for around 40% of all nosocomial infections reported to the Center for Disease Control and Prevention (CDC) in the USA, with prevalence varying between 1 and 10% (WONG; HOOTON, 1981). It can be seen that the situation is no different in developing countries and that UTIs are also one of the main causes of hospital-acquired infections. According to a multicentre cross-sectional prevalence study in Turkey, 16% of urinary tract infections were analysed, followed by ventilator-associated pneumonia and bloodstream infections (ESEN; LEBLEBICIOGLU, 2004).

Women are more vulnerable than men to developing a urinary tract infection. Adult women are 50 times more likely to acquire a UTI than men and 30% of women experience symptomatic UTI during their lifetime. Because the main route of contamination of the urinary tract is via the ascending route, women have a smaller anatomical extension of the urethra and greater proximity between the vagina and the anus, which are characteristics of the female genitalia (MASSON et al., 2009).

Although it occurs more commonly in women, the incidence of UTI is higher among men over 50 (HEAD, 2008). Instrumentation of the urinary tract, including bladder catheterisation, and the occurrence of prostate disease are conditions involved in the incidence in men (LOPES; TAVARES, 2004). Among the elderly and hospitalised individuals, UTI rates are also high for the reasons mentioned above and for the presence of comorbidities that increase susceptibility to infections (LOPES; TAVARES, 2004).

Urinary infection can take two forms: symptomatic or asymptomatic. And in terms of localisation, it can be determined as low or high. UTI can simply affect the lower urinary tract, identifying the diagnosis of cystitis, or it can affect both the lower and upper urinary tracts, characterising upper urinary tract infection, known as pyelonephritis (LOPES; TAVARES, 2004).

The causes of urinary retention can be congenital or acquired (LUCCHETTI et al., 2005). Congenital UTIs are characterised by narrowing of the meatus in boys and, in girls, the valves of the posterior urethra and the ureterovesical and ureteropelvic junctions. Acquired UTIs are most frequently caused by neurogenic bladder, prostatism, ureteral calculi, fibrosis or malignant retroperitoneal tumours and pregnancy (MERMEL, 2000).

Among UTIs, those that affect patients who chronically use bladder catheters are of paramount importance (MERMEL, 2000). These patients have difficulty eliminating urine and, consequently, urinary retention which, if not treated properly, can lead to numerous other complications (KUNIN, 1997).

During invasive procedures with bladder catheterisation, the patient is more prone to acquiring urinary tract infections. Thus, the development of infection depends on multiple factors involved in the bacteria-host relationship. Bacterial factors (virulence and adherence to urothelial receptors) (STAMM, 1991), host factors (normal bacterial flora, acidic vaginal pH, urinary pH, high urea concentration, organic acids, act of urination), genetic factors and anatomo-functional alterations to the urinary tract normally make it difficult for uropathogens to adhere to the urothelium and are reduced (NETO, 1999). In addition to these factors, asepsis and bladder catheterisation techniques and catheterisation time also influence the increase in urinary infection rates (LUCCHETTI et al., 2005).

3.   3Candida spp.

The genus Candida belongs to the kingdom Fungi, group Eumycota, phylum Deuteromycota, class Blastomycetes and is part of the family Cryptococcacea (COLOMBO; GUIMARÃES, 2003). It has around 163 species and

approximately 10 are responsible for infections in humans (CASTRO et al., 2006).

Infections caused by yeasts of the genus Candida are of great importance due to the high frequency with which they infect and colonise the host, representing a growing threat to human health. The incidence of infections by these microorganisms has increased significantly over the last 20 years. Some factors predetermine Candida infection, such as the use of prostheses, probes, catheters, endotracheal tubes and pacemakers. These devices facilitate the colonisation of these microorganisms, allowing biofilms to form (WINGETER et al., 2007).

The general characteristics of yeasts of the genus Candida are: eukaryotic microorganisms devoid of photosynthesising pigments that have a cell wall consisting mainly of chitin and a phospholipid plasma membrane that has various sterols, with ergosterol predominating. Their nutrition comes from carbon sources soaked up from the environment, as a result of their rigid cell wall which does not allow phagocytosis to take place (AGUIAR, 2007).

Only 10% of yeasts are recognised as etiological agents in human infections, which are usually determined as opportunistic commensals on the surface of mucous membranes and skin (VALLE et al., 2010). As for the C. albicans species, it represents around 60 to 90 per cent of isolations, C. tropicalis 7 per cent, and other species such as C. krusei, C. guillermondii, C. glabrata and C. parapsilosis are less common (MAGDALENA; PERRONE, 2001; LACAZ, 1980; MARTINS et al., 2002; RIBEIRO, 2002; SCHERMA et al., 2004; URIZAR, 2002).

The commensal fungus Candida spp. is present in the microbiota, inhabiting places such as the oral cavity, gastrointestinal tract, vagina and skin of healthy individuals (COLOMBO et al., 2006). Species of the genus Candida have been the most common agents of

These isolates account for around 80% of hospital-acquired fungal infections and are the fourth leading cause of bloodstream infection, leading to death in around 25% to 38% of patients who develop candidemia (TAMURA et al., 2007).

The most relevant species is Candida albicans due to its prevalence in both healthy and immune compromised hosts (VALLE et al., 2010; BARBEDO; SGARBI, 2010; SUZUKI, 2009). This yeast is found abundantly in nature, occupying various habitats, unlike other species of the genus with a more restricted distribution (ÁLVARES et al., 2007).

In terms of microbiological aspects, Candida albicans is initially defined by its moist colonial morphology, specific and creamy odour, smooth or rough appearance and yellowish-white colour in Sabouraud agar culture medium, germ tube production, carbon assimilation and fermentative competence. For its growth to be favoured, it must be found at temperatures ranging from 20°C to 38°C. Acidic pH helps their proliferation, with the ideal pH range being between 2.5 and 7.5. Microscopically, yeast cells have a spherical, ovoid or elongated shape, measuring around 3 to 5μm in diameter and are Gram-positive in preparations stained using this technique (RIBEIRO, 2008; ANDRADE, 2006; BARBIERI, 2005).

Candida albicans is a commensal yeast found naturally in the oral mucosa, urogenital tract, gastrointestinal tract and skin of human beings from birth onwards, due to exceptional circumstances when there is a disruption in the biological balance as a result of predisposing factors (physiological, pathological, mechanical and immunological), and an increase in the multiplication and invasion of tissues by these microorganisms may occur, giving rise to infections known as candidiasis (VALLE et al., 2010; MARTINS et al., 2002; SUZUKI, 2009).

This yeast is adapted to the human body and can colonise it, thus not generating signs of disease (ÁLVARES et al., 2007; RIBEIRO et al., 2007). This balance between Candida and the host is due to the maintenance of the integrity of the tissue barriers, the harmonious relationship between the autochthonous microbiota and the proper functioning of the human immune system. On the other hand, the fungus displays its ability to adhere and produce enzymes and toxins in a balanced way (CALDERONE; FONZIWA, 2001; VIEIRA et al., 2005).

The virulence causes of C. albicans increase its effectiveness in developing mucosal or systemic infections, depending on the stage and nature of the host response. Commonly, these infectious processes benefit from the disruption of the parasite-host balance. The main factors of this fungus that characterise its ability to colonise and then cause infection are: polymorphism, production of extracellular enzymes, phenotypic variability and toxins (RIBEIRO, 2008).

Both the infectious process and colonisation begin with the adherence of the yeast to the epithelial cells. The presence of specific receptors on the cytoplasmic membrane is necessary for the penetration and intracellular fixation of the fungus (MAGDALENA; PERRONE, 2001). As for adhesion to the host's cell surfaces, this is influenced by factors such as the availability of carbohydrates, germ tube formation, temperature, pH, production of phospholipases, other extracellular enzymes and proteases (VIDOTTO et al., 2003).

It can be said that the adhesion of Candida cells is, however, a complex and multifactorial phenomenon that consists of the expression of various types of adhesins on the surfaces of morphologically altered cells. This is in addition to the ability to form a biofilm on host cells, which is a defining characteristic of this pathogen, resulting in stable attachment of the fungus to tissues (KHAN et al., 2010).

This adherence mechanism involves glycoproteins, lectin-like proteins that can distinguish various types of sugar and receptors for the C3b fraction of the complement system. On the host side, there are cell receptors for Candida adhesins such as fibronectin, fibrin and laminin, which benefit colonisation of the extracellular matrix (RIBEIRO, 2008).

Biofilm can develop on both biological surfaces and inert surfaces such as catheters. Biofilm formation is important in the pathogenicity of Candida because it makes it a barrier against the penetration of host immunological factors and antimicrobial drugs (VUONG et al., 2004). This occurs due to the formation of a polysaccharide extracellular matrix, which inhibits the diffusion of antimicrobial molecules into the biofilm, or due to the ionic action of the biofilm, which reduces its expected action (COSTA et al., 2013).

3.4 Microbial biofilm

Various microorganisms are found in nature as communities attached to certain biofilm surfaces. This microbial growth has profound effects on the environment, industry and human health (HALL- STOODLEY et al., 2004). The term biofilm was introduced in 1978 by Costerton and colleagues, but it was Antonie van Leuuwenhoek who, at the beginning of the 7th century, first observed the formation of a biofilm on his own teeth (SINGH et al., 2015; VASUDEVAN, 2014).

Biofilms are aggregates of microorganisms embedded in a polymeric matrix and adhered to a solid surface, forming a porous and highly hydrated structure containing exopolysaccharides (EPS) and small channels open between microcolonies (LAWRENCE et al., 1991). This type of organisation is extremely advantageous for all species of microorganisms as it provides protection against adversities such as dehydration, colonisation by bacteriophages and resistance to antimicrobials (GILBERT et al., 2003).

Biofilm development is an ancient form of prokaryote adaptation (HALL-STOODLEY et al., 2004). It represents a mode of development that allows bacteria to survive in hostile environments and to colonise new places through the mechanism of dispersal (HALL-STOODLEY; STOODLEY, 2005; PUREVDORJ-GAJE et al., 2005; MAI-PROCHNOW et al., 2008).

Biofilms formed by bacteria show coordinated behaviour by building complex three-dimensional structures and bacterial communities that are functionally heterogeneous (STOODLEY et al., 2002; HALL-STOODLEY et al., 2004). This phenotypic heterogeneity or specialisation present in biofilms is impressive. For example, it can be said that bacterial populations in biofilms exhibit differences in the expression of surface molecules, nutrient utilisation, antibiotic resistance and virulence factors (BAGGE et al., 2004; VOUNG et al., 2004; PEARSON et al., 2006; JURCISEK; BAKALETZ, 2007; LENZ et al., 2008; ZHANG; MAH, 2008).

Urinary tract infection (UTI) is one of the main types of hospital-acquired infection, and the presence of a urinary catheter is the main risk factor (PLOWMAN et al., 2001; KALSI et al., 2003). There are other risk factors associated with bacteriuria in catheterised patients, including the duration of the procedure, type of catheterisation and drainage system, antimicrobial therapy, severity of the condition that led to hospitalisation and underlying disease (KALSI et al., 2003; LEONE et al., 2003).

Urinary tract infections occur more frequently in women due to certain factors intrinsic to the female apparatus when compared to the male apparatus, such as: extension of the urethra and colonisation of the periurethral region (MIMS et al., 2000). Among the risk factors, urinary tract infections and the use of urinary catheters have been considered the most important for the development of bacteriuria (LUCCHETTI et al., 2005).

Since Candida albicans is capable of invading practically all body sites, including deep tissues and organs, superficial sites such as nails, mucous membranes and skin. As for superficial infections, acute pseudomembranous infections of the vaginal or oral cavity are the most common (ANDES et al., 2004; BENNETT et al., 2003). Biomaterials such as stents, shunts, prostheses (valve, voice, knee, cardiac, among others), endotracheal tubes, pacemakers and catheters also contribute to the colonisation and formation of biofilms by Candida (NOBILE et al., 2006).

For colonisation, the yeast cells must first adhere to the host cells and to the tissues or surfaces of the biomaterial that are wrapped with a conditioning film of glycoproteins (NOBILE et al., 2006). This conditioning film is produced on the surface of biomaterials and tissue substrates immediately after implantation, because biomedical devices are usually surrounded by body fluids such as blood, urine, synovial fluid and saliva (NOBILE et al., 2006).

A characteristic of C. albicans biofilms is that they usually consist of a mixture of morphological forms (BAILLIE; DOUGLAS, 1999). On catheter discs and plastic surfaces, the C. albicans biofilm has two layers: a thin base layer of yeast cells covered by a thicker but more open hyphal layer (CHANDRA et al., 2001).

3.5 Resistance   to antifungal drugs

Recently, the isolation of yeast strains with reduced susceptibility or resistance to antifungal drugs has been frequently observed. The resistance of microorganisms to antifungals, in vitro or clinically, has occurred when the cells of susceptible fungi are exposed to previous contact with the drug or is a characteristic of the microorganism (SILVA et al., 2002).

The first hypothesis can be said to be the result of low levels of the drug in the blood and tissue, due to interaction between the drugs or the patient's immunodepression. In vitro resistance, on the other hand, must be of secondary origin, where susceptible strains become resistant due to previous contact with the antifungal. It is understood that this drug resistance is dependent on contact between the host, the drug and the fungus, but one of the most important factors in the emergence of resistance is the patient's condition (SILVA et al., 2002).

As in the case of azole agents, they interfere with the biosynthesis of ergosterol, the sterol found in large quantities in the plasma membrane of fungi. The action of these drugs is due to the inhibition of the enzyme 14a- demethylase (14 DM), a cytochrome P 450 enzyme important in the ergosterol biosynthesis pathway, which catalyses the oxidative removal of the 14a-methyl group from lanosterol. Azole agents that are bound to the active site of 14 DM compete with the substrate for binding (KELLY et al., 1993).

Modifications in the sterol biosynthesis pathway and the high expression of the ERG 11 gene, involved in the synthesis of the 14 DM enzyme, may modify the development of resistance in Candida sp. In the case of fluconazole, mutations in the ERG 11 gene result in a decreased affinity of 14 DM to it, thus reducing the intracellular accumulation of the drug and its inactivation, leading to a progression of the microorganism's resistance (MORSCHHÀUSER, 2002). The blocking of 14 DM by fluconazole results from a decrease in ergosterol and the accumulation of a methylated sterol, 14α-methylergoste-8,24, dien-3β, 6α-diol, which inhibits cell development. Modifications in sterol biosynthesis can prevent the accumulation of this growth inhibitor and define resistance to fluconazole

(MORSCHHÀUSER, 2002; MUNOZ et al., 2002).

As drug resistance among Candida spp. has been one of the aggravating problems, the use of susceptibility tests in clinical isolations has become essential. Prior recognition of the Candida species and definition of in vitro susceptibility have been recommended in certain cases, such as oropharyngeal candidiasis in HIV-infected patients, recurrent vaginitis and systemic mycoses (ZARDO; MEZZARI, 2004).

In the day-to-day life of the mycology laboratory, it is necessary to adapt methods that help to assess antifungal susceptibility, due to the high resistance of yeasts, resulting in a reduction in the therapeutic amount available (LOPES et al., 2001). Being aware of drug sensitivity makes it possible to optimise treatment (COLOMBO et al., 1999).

3.6 Essential oils

Essential oils are extracted from plants using vapour drag techniques or by pressing the pericarp of citrus fruits. They are complex mixtures of volatile, lipophilic, generally odourous and liquid substances resulting from the secondary metabolism of plants. Their composition can contain 100 or more organic compounds belonging to the most diverse classes, with terpenes and phenylpropenes being the most commonly found (CASTRO et al., 2004). They are mainly composed of mono- and sesquiterpenes and phenylpropanoids, metabolites that confer organoleptic characteristics (BIZZO et al., 2009).

These aromatic products are produced by secretory cells or groups of cells found in some parts of the plant, such as stems and leaves.

They are present in certain areas of the plant, such as leaves, fruit or bark, in different concentrations (CONNER, 2003). The use of essential oils stands out due to their prospective functionalities, as they contain compounds that are used in the pharmaceutical perfumery industry to create natural remedies, prototypes of pharmacologically active substances, food formulations and sanitisers, due to the wide public acceptance of natural products (SIMÕES et al., 2001; SCHERER et al., 2009).

According to the literature, numerous reports highlight the biological activity of plant extracts, including antifungal, antibacterial, anti-inflammatory, analgesic, antitumour and antioxidant activity (SCHERER et al., 2009). Essential oils have long served as the basis for various applications in folk medicine, including the production of topical antiseptics. This has served as the basis for various scientific investigations aimed at confirming their antimicrobial activity (ALMEIDA et al., 2006; ARRUDA et al., 2006; NUNES et al 2006; BENKEBLIA, 2004; REHDER et al., 2004; CLAFFEY, 2003; SEYMOUR, 2003; ARWEILER et al., 2000; FINE et al., 2000; PAN et al., 2000). Where this antimicrobial action is presented in three ways: interference in the phospholipid double layer of the bacterial cell wall, increased permeability and loss of cellular constituents, and alteration of a variety of enzyme systems such as those involved in cellular energy production and synthesis of structural components or destruction of genetic material (SIQUEIRA et al., 2015).

The resurgence of interest in natural therapies and the increase in consumption of effective and safe natural products calls for more studies and data on plant oils and extracts (DE-SOUZA et al., 2006; OLIVEIRA et al., 2006; LIS-BACHIN; DEANS, 1997).

With regard to the antimicrobial activity of essential oils, in vitro tests there is a diversity of methodologies proposed, making it problematic to compare these studies (HAMMER et al., 1999). The methods normally used are disc diffusion, diffusion using cavities made in agar, dilution in agar and dilution in broth to determine the minimum inhibitory concentration (MIC) (NOSTRO et al., 2004; CIMANGA et al., 2002; SHAFI et al., 2002; CANILLAC; MOUREY, 2001; TAKAISI-KIKUNI et al., 2000). The results obtained with each method used can differ due to factors such as the changes between tests with regard to microbial growth, the display of microorganisms in the oil, the solubility of the oil or its constituents and the use and quantity of emulsifier (OPALCHENOVA; OBRESHKOVA, 2003; HOOD et al., 2003; LAMBERT et al., 2001; HAMMER et al., 1999).

There is an interest in broadening knowledge about the inhibitory concentrations of essential oils, in search of stability between acceptability and the effectiveness of antimicrobial action. The MIC can be determined in in vitro and in vivo studies. The methods available can be divided into: diffusion, impedance, dilution and optical density (TASSOU et al., 2000). Of these, the dilution method has proved to be the most effective, providing quantitative data, while diffusion in a Petri dish is a qualitative method, which is why these methods (dilution and diffusion) are not necessarily comparable. The results achieved by each of these methods may differ due to factors intrinsic to the tests (NASCIMENTO et al., 2007).

As for the particularities of the oil, some research has shown that even intra-specific genetic variations in the plant species can modify the content of the active ingredient in the oil. What's more, other factors such as climate, season, soil and planting method, use of pesticides, fertilisation, irrigation, environmental conditions and weather, extraction technique, origin of the plant material (fresh or dried), botanical source, harvesting and cultivation and geographical variation patterns (latitudes and longitudes) can affect the chemical composition of the oils, which can cause changes in antimicrobial activity (SEFIDKON et al., 2007; APEL et al., 2006; ASEKUN et al., 2006; CARVALHO-FILHO et al., 2006; OLIVEIRA et al., 2005; POTZERNHEIM et al., 2006; TELCI et al., 2006; FRANCO et al.., 2005; VILJOEN et al., 2005; BASSOLE et al., 2003; OPALCHENOVA; OBRESHKOVA, 2003; AZEVEDO et al., 2002; RASSOLI; MIRMOSTAFA, 2002; LAMBERT et al., 2001).

3.7 Palmarosa oil

Palmarosa (Cymbopogon martini) is a plant belonging to the Poacea family, native to India and cultivated on a large scale, especially in tropical and subtropical regions (LORENZI, 2002; PATTNAIK et al., 1997; VAN ZYL et al., 2006; DUARTE et al., 2007; JIROVETZ et al., 2007). It is a very aromatic grass species, where its essential oil is popularly used as a raw material for perfumes, soaps, floral pink perfumes, cosmetic preparations, used to mask the odour of botanical pesticides and in the manufacture of mosquito repellents. In medicine, its oil is used against ageing and dry skin, to relieve stress and in compresses for cramps (RAO et al., 2005).

Palmarosa essential oil is rich in geraniol (70-90%), with other chemical compounds being (E)-β-ocimene, linalool, geranyl acetate and β-caryophyllene, depending on the botanical material and the method of extracting the essential oil (RAO; RAO; PUTTANNA,

2001; KHANUJA et al., 2005). The chemical composition of the essential oil can vary due to genetic diversity, habitat and cultivation. Another important factor for high productivity of essential oil rich in active ingredients is the choice of genotype (LEAL et al., 2001).

Because the main constituent of palmarosa is geraniol, which is a monoterpenoid and an alcohol, it has different pharmacological properties, including efficacy against insects, anti-tumour, anti-infectious, immunomodulatory and antimicrobial activity, such as against C. albicans (ATCC 10231), S. aureus, E. coli and S. Thyphimurium (SHERER et al., 2009; ALMEIDA et al., 2011; PATTNAIK et al., 1997; VAN ZYL et al., 2006; DUARTE et al., 2007; JIROVETZ et al., 2007).

According to some studies on the action of geraniol on Candida cells, these showed that when observed under a scanning electron microscope, Candida cells showed their morphology altered in the presence of geraniol. According to them, the cells were broken or wrinkled, while the untreated cells were intact. Geraniol altered the sterol pattern of Candida species, completely blocking ergosterol which is an essential component of the fungal cytoplasmic membrane (SHARMA et al., 2016).

CHAPTER 4

METHODOLOGY

4.1   Study site

The study was carried out in the Pharmaceutical Technology and Microbiology laboratories at the Integrated Regional University of Alto Uruguay and the Missions (URI) in Santiago.

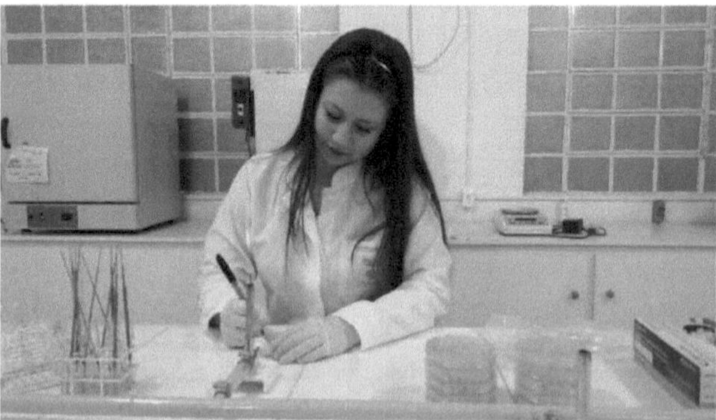

Figure 1: Microbiology Laboratory.

4.2   Purchase of palmarosa oil

Palmarosa oil (OP) was purchased from the company Phitoterápica, batch POEP17.02, valid until 04/19 (São Paulo, Brazil).

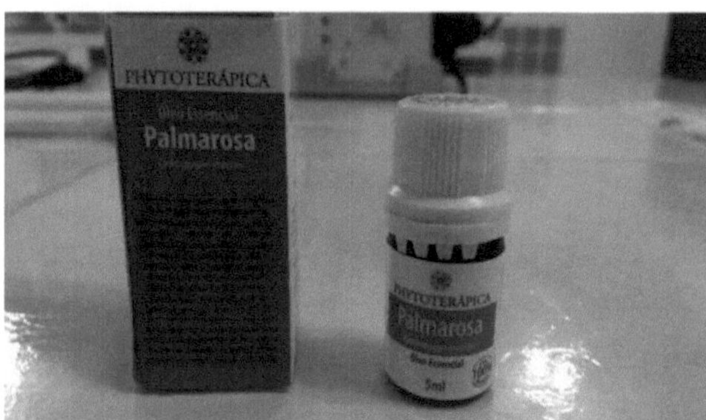

Figure 2: Palmarosa oil from the Phitoterápica company.

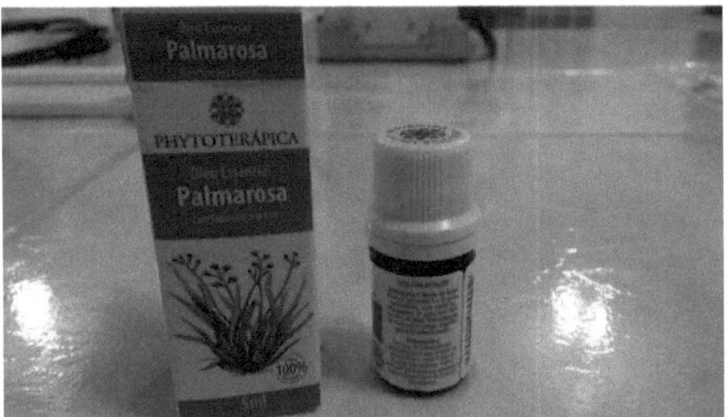

Figure 3: Palmarosa oil from the Phitoterápica company.

4.3 Gas Chromatography - Mass Spectrometry (GC-MS)

GC-MS analyses were carried out on an Agilent Technologies Autosystem XL GC-MS, operating without El Mode at 70 eV, equipped with a split/splitless injector (250 °C). The transfer line temperature was 280°C. Helium was used as the carrier gas (1.5mL/min) and capillary columns were a 5MS HP (30m x 0.25mm; thickness make film 0.25mm) and an Innowax HP (30m x 0.32mm id, thickness make film 0.50mm). The temperature programme was the same. The volume injected was 1 ul of oil (GIONGO et al., 2016).

4. 4 Substrates

The substrates used for biofilm adhesion were sterile polyurethane urinary catheters (GIONGO et al., 2016).

4. 5 Biofilm formation and treatment

Suspensions of C. albicans ATCC 14053, adjusted to the McFarland 1.0 turbidity scale, were used to form the biofilms. A biofilm formation control was carried out for each plate, inoculated with each species of microorganism added to BHI broth (Brain Heart Infusion Broth, Himedia®) (GIONGO et al, 2016).

The experiments with urinary catheters were carried out after cutting them into 3 cm fragments. These were placed in previously sterilised tubes (11 x 11 cm) containing 4 mL of

BHI broth. Subsequently, 1 mL of C. albicans suspension was added to each tube and incubated at 35 ± 2°C for 10 days for biofilm formation. This formation was monitored daily and the culture medium in the tubes was replaced when necessary. After formation, the Candida sp. biofilms were treated with 1 mL of palmarosa oil, determined by the MIC of 1/8 at a concentration of 110 μg/mL-1, which showed antifungal activity, and were incubated again at 35 ± 2°C for 72 hours. After this period, the probes were washed three times with sterile water to remove the planktonic cells and transferred to new tubes to carry out the quantification tests (GIONGO et al., 2016).

4.6Quantification of the biofilm

Quantification was carried out in order to estimate the number of fungi present in the biofilms and the amount that would remain after treatment with the samples. The classic method of counting CFU/mL on agar (carried out for the urinary tube) was used. Briefly, in order to carry out this quantification, the biofilms present on the probes after the treatments were duly scraped off using a sterile needle, washed with 1 mL of physiological solution and collected in a 1.5 mL microtube. Each treatment was inoculated using a calibrated loop (10 μL) on BHI agar, and the plates were incubated at 35 ± 2°C for 48 hours. The colonies were counted and the results expressed in CFU/mL (GIONGO et al., 2016).

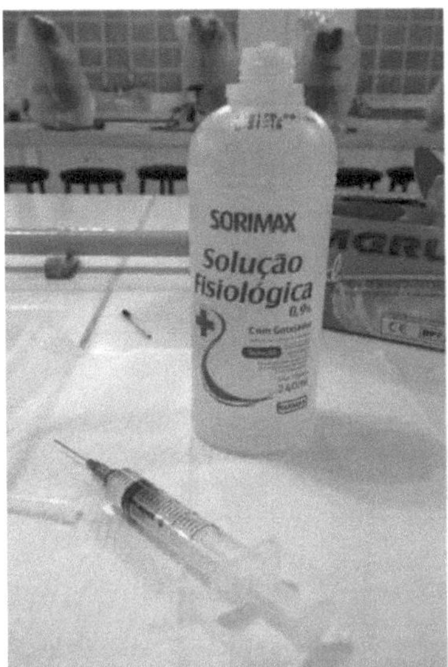

Figure 4: Physiological solution and sterile needle used.

4.   7Statistical analysis

All tests were carried out in triplicate with mean and standard deviation (SD).

CHAPTER 5

RESULTS AND DISCUSSIONS

Palmarosa oil was analysed using gas chromatography. Three main constituents were identified: geraniol (35.27%), neral (13.09%) and geranyl acetate (9.68%). The total characterisation results are shown in **Table 1**.

Table 1. Composition of Palmarosa Essential Oil.

Components	IR[a]	Palmarosa	
		IR[b]	(%)[c]
0-Myrcene	991	989	1.71
p-Cimene	1026	1027	5.82
Linalool	1098	1099	2.09
Camphenol	1109	1112	0.65
Nerol	1228	1228	1.83
Neral	1240	1141	13.09
Geraniol	1255	1253	35.27
Carvacrol	1298	1296	0.45
E-Citral	1341	1341	3.17
Geranyl acetate	1383	1380	9.68
0-Elemene	1391	1388	4.35
0-Caryophyllene	1418	1419	5.92
Neryl propanate	1454	1459	1.69
Aromandrene	1461	1460	0.81
Valencene	1491	1489	0.36
(Z)-Nerolidol	1534	1533	1.57
Elemol	1549	1550	0.29
Geranyl butyrate	1562	1561	1.63
Caryophyllene oxide	1581	1580	2.79
Globulol	1583	1585	0.91
Viridiflorol	1590	1593	1.13
(E,E)-Famesol	1722	1725	4.52
Total identified (%)			**99.73**

aRetention rates from the literature (Adams, 1995).
bExperimental retention indices (based on C7-C30 n-alkane homologous series).
cRelative proportions of essential oil components were expressed as percentages.

After carrying out the gas chromatography of palmarosa oil, what had already been shown in several studies was confirmed: geraniol is the main constituent present in the oil. According to (PRASHAR et al., 2003; CHEN; VILJOEN, 2010; MALLAVARAPU et al..,

1998), this acyclic alcoholic monoterpene constituent is a mixture of two isomers, geraniol (trans) and nerol (cis), found in various essential oils, including palmarosa oil (Cymbopogon martini) (53.5%-65%), wild bergamot (Monarda fistulosa) (>95%), ninde oil (66.0%), rose oil (44.4%) and citronella oil (24.8%).

Geraniol is emitted by flowers of various species and is present in vegetative tissues. It often coexists as geranial and neral, which are its oxidation products. So the main registered constituents of interest are: Geranyl acetate, Linalool and β-Caryophyllene, although variations occur in the composition in different extractions depending on the oil extraction method and the plant material (CHEN; VILJOEN, 2010; PRASHAR et al., 2003).

In this study, the minimum inhibitory concentration of palmarosa oil against Candida albicans was determined, as shown in Table 2. The following oil concentrations were used: 442 μL mL^{-1} , 221 μL mL^{-1} , 110.5 μL mL^{-1} , 55.25 μL mL^{-1} , 27.62 μL mL^{-1} . It was found that up to a concentration of 110.5 μg/mL^{-1} the oil inhibited the growth of Candida albicans strains. Thus, the result obtained showed that in small concentrations the oil is capable of acting as an antifungal.

Studies have shown the importance of the main constituent of palmarosa oil (Cymbopogon martini), which has antifungal action, being fungistatic against filamentous fungi Aspergillus niger, Chaetomium globosum and Penicillium funiculosum, and also possessing antimicrobial properties (PRASHAR et al., 2003; DELESPAUL et al., 2000; SHARMA et al., 2016). Other studies looking for constituents that have antifungal therapeutic potential include, as an example of a vegetative product, the essential oil of tulsi, whose active components are Eugenol, Linalool and Citral, which have been shown to have antifungal activity (SHARMA et al., 2016).

Table 2: Antifungal activity of Cymbopogon Martini **essential oil (MIC) against** Candida albicans **using the macrodilution method.**

Microorganism	Palmarosa oil (MIC)
Candida albicans	110.5 p,g/mL^{-1}

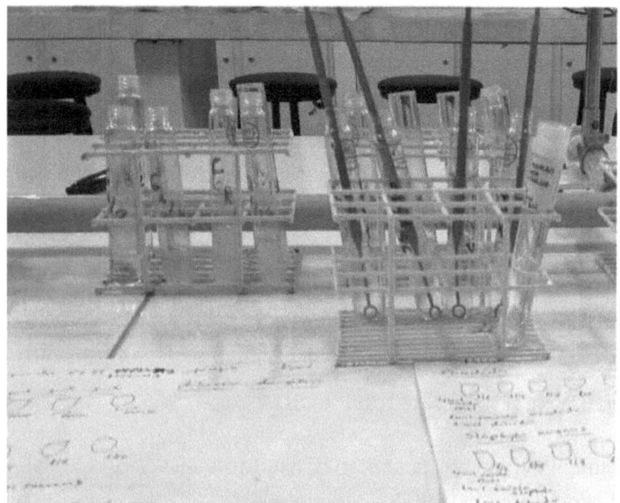

Figure 5: Determining the MIC using the macrodilution method.

Researchers have demonstrated how antifungal activity works against Candida albicans, such as the activity of azoles, which inhibit sterol 14-demethylase, whose inhibition is correlated with the cessation of cell growth; because ergosterol is the main sterol component of fungal cell membranes, being essential for normal cell growth, and among other functions, becoming vital for survival (SHARMA et al., 2016). Thus, authors indicate that geraniol has a fungicidal rather than fungistatic action, being correlated with the inhibition of ergosterol content; due to its effect on the proton pumping of H+-ATPase located in the plasma membrane, thus disrupting the integrity of the cell membrane and homeostasis (SHARMA et al., 2016), The main objective of this study was to evaluate the inhibitory potential of Cymbopogon martini oil, more popularly known as palmarosa, on biofilms formed by strains of Candida albicans ATCC 14053 adhered to urinary catheters. Figure 6 below shows the formation of C. albicans biofilms on urinary catheters.

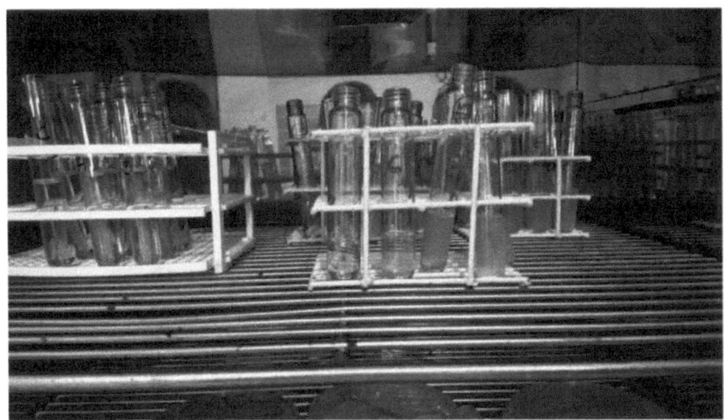

Figure 6: Biofilm formation on urinary catheters stored in an oven at 35°C.

Table 3 shows the formation of Candida albicans biofilm on hospital medical equipment. A control was carried out to check the adherence of the biofilm to the urinary catheters.

Table 3: Control of Candida albicans **biofilm formation.**

Samples	CFU/mL
Control + Control -	1.08 x 10³ CFU mL *⁻¹

Control +: probe, BHI broth, inoculum. Control -: probe and BHI broth. * No growth

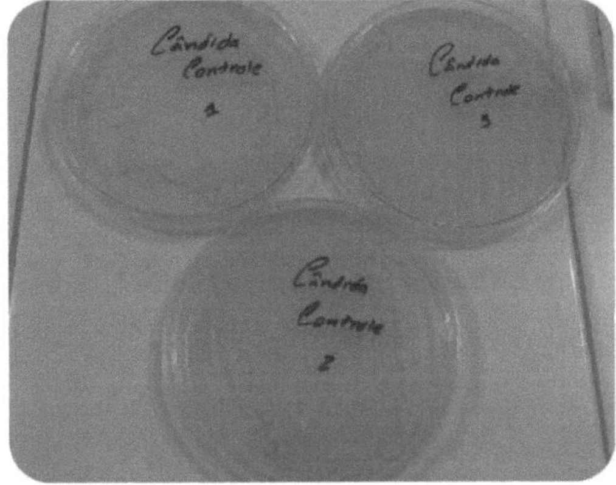

Figure 7: Positive control.

The search for new alternatives to combat these resistant microorganisms has only increased, as the resistance of Candida species to synthetic antifungals, such as the drug resistance of C. albicans to azole derivatives, has become a serious problem (ALMEIDA et al., 2011). Including its ability to adhere to hospital materials due to biofilm formation, which increases its virulence or pathogenicity (ALMEIDA et al., 2011). The use of natural products has therefore been emphasised with a view to obtaining better performance and efficacy against these microorganisms (JANTAM et al., 2008; LIMA et al., 2006; POZZATTI, 2008).

According to (CEGELSKI et al., 2008), the term biofilm refers to the attachment to surfaces of microbial communities contained in self-produced extracellular polymerisation matrices. In in vitro systems, different types of synthetic materials are used for adhesion and biofilm formation, such as plastics, silicones and metals, since insertion into these substrates is the result of physical and chemical interactions between the cell surface and the substrate (COAD et al., 2014; NWAUGO et al 2007; CHANDRA et al., 2001; WEBB et al., 1999). Thus, in bacteria and C. albicans, hydrophobic interactions and electrostatic forces are responsible for the initial binding to these surfaces (KIPANGA; LUYTEN, 2017; VARGHESE et al., 1999; DONLAN, 2002).The results obtained were satisfactory. Treatment with palmarosa oil proved to be effective, demonstrating the existence of antibiofilm activity. Treatment with the solvent DMSO was also carried out to demonstrate that it does not interfere with the development of the biofilm, as C. albicans grew.

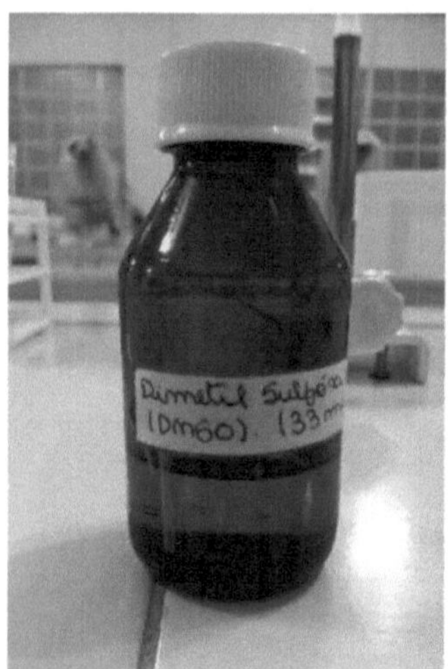

Figure 8: DMSO solvent.

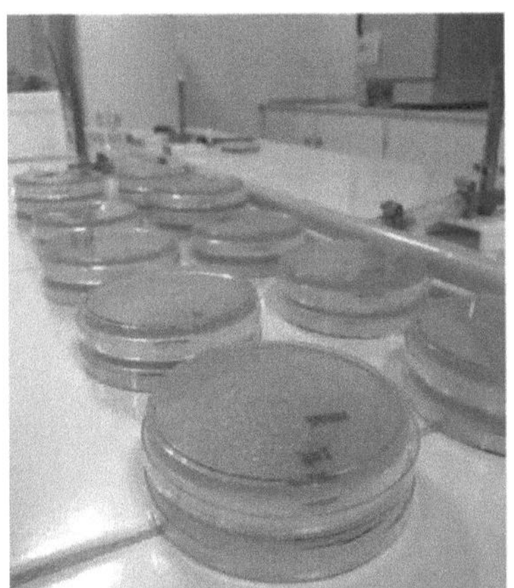

Figura 9: Plates.

Figure 10 shows the biofilm formation of the samples in urinary catheters, and Table 4 shows the CFU/mL values.

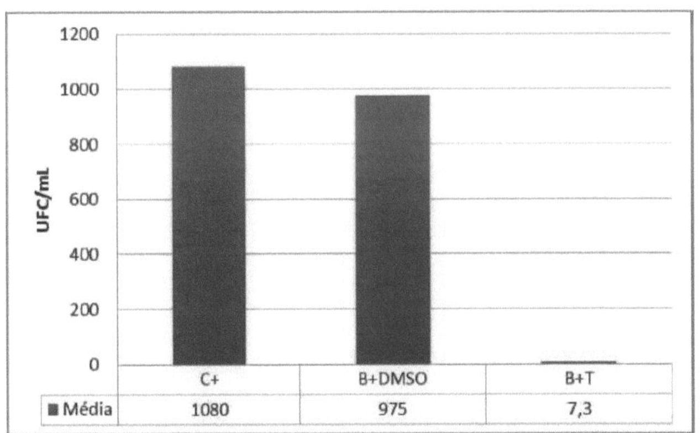

Figura 10:   Graph showing the formation of biofilm on urinary tube samples.

C+: probe, BHI broth, inoculum. B + DMSO: probe, BHI broth, inoculum, DMSO. B + T: probe, BHI broth, inoculum,
DMSO, palmarosa oil.

Table 4: CFU/mL values and standard deviation.

Samples	CFU/mL±SD
Control +	1.08×10^3 UFCmL^{-1} + 73.54
Biofilm + DMSO	0.97×10^3 UFCmL^{-1} + 38.18
Biofilm + Treatment	$0.007 \times 10_3$ CFU mL^{-1} + 1.15

Control +: probe, BHI broth, inoculum. Biofilm + DMSO: probe, BHI broth, inoculum, DMSO. Biofilm +

Treatment: probe, BHI broth, inoculum, DMSO, palmarosa oil.

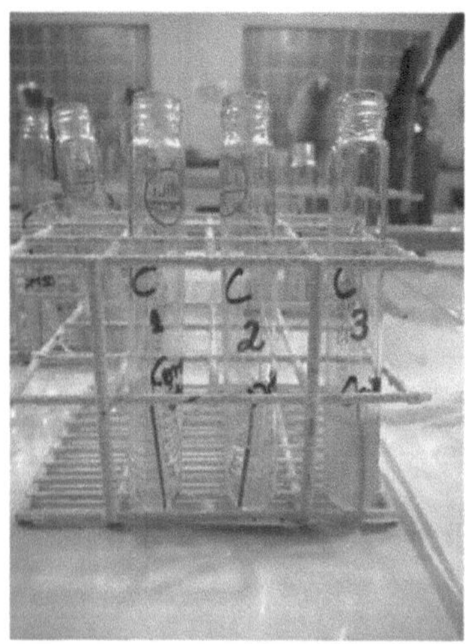

Figura 11:   C + Treatment, C + DMSO and C + BHI Broth.

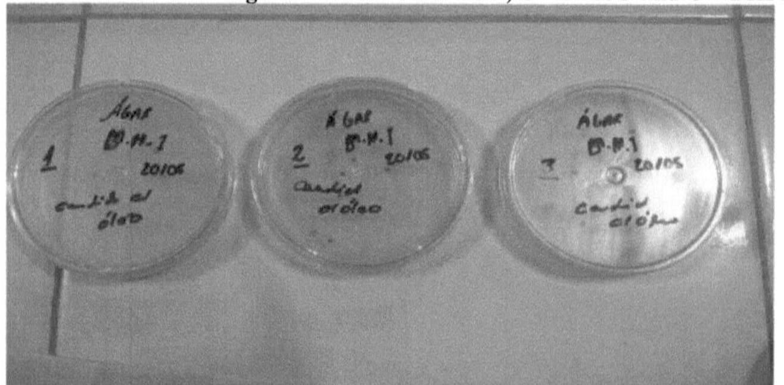

Figure 12: Palmarosa oil treatment.

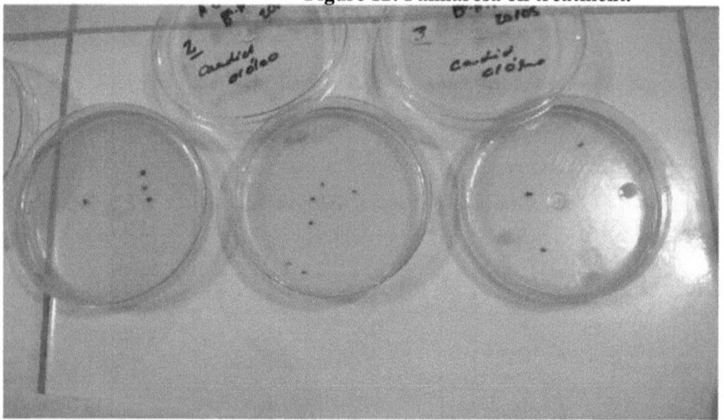

Figure 13: Palmarosa oil treatment.

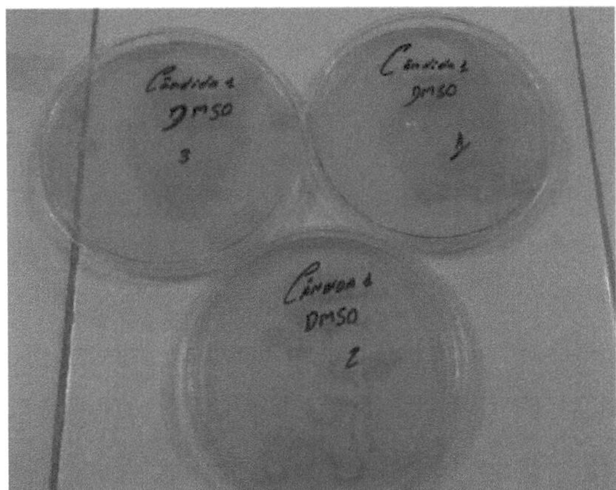

Figure 14: Treatment with DMSO.

The antifungal action of this oil against Candida albicans strains and its antibiofilm activity could be observed in this study. It can be concluded that the palmarosa oil (Cymbopogon martini) used to treat biofilm is effective, because when the CFU/mL count was carried out, a low growth rate of C. albicans strains was observed. There are not many reports and studies on the antibiofilm activity of palmarosa oil, but this study has already shown that this action is extremely important and of interest in the fight against these resistant microorganisms and in reducing hospital infection rates.

CHAPTER 6

CONCLUSION

Palmarosa oil has some very interesting constituents, but the main one, which is found in large quantities, is geraniol. It has a number of important properties, such as its antifungal action, which is extremely important in the fight against resistant microorganisms in the hospital environment. With the power of Candida albicans to adhere to urinary catheters, its degree of resistance to antifungal drugs is high, so interest in new alternatives to combat it has increased. There are no studies in the literature on the antibiofilm activity of Palmorosa oil, but the effectiveness of the antifungal action prevailed against C. albicans.

In this study, the tests carried out confirmed the antifungal activity of Cymbopogon martini essential oil against strains of C. albicans. The treatment of C. albicans biofilm with palmarosa oil showed significant results, demonstrating that this oil has antibiofilm activity. Although there have not been many studies and reports on antibiofilm action, this research shows that this activity has been detected, demonstrating its importance when used to combat resistant microorganisms and reduce hospital infection rates.

REFERENCES

AGUIAR, Michelle Maria Gonçalves Barão de. **Development of New Nystatin Oral Tablets for the Treatment of Oral Candidiasis**. 2007.146 f. Dissertation (Master's Degree in Pharmaceutical Sciences) - Faculty of Pharmacy, Federal University of Rio de Janeiro, Rio de Janeiro, 2007.

ALMEIDA, J.R.G.A.; SILVA-FILHO, R.N.; NUNES, X.P.; DIAS, C.S.; PEREIRA, F.O.; LIMA, E.O. Antimicrobial activity of the essential oil of Bowdichia virgiloides Kunt. **Rev Bras Farmacogn**. v. 16, p. 638-641, 2006.

ALMEIDA, L.; CALVALCANTI, Y.; VIANA, W.; LIMA, E. Screening of the Antifungal Activity of Essential Oils on Candida albicans. **Brazilian Journal of Health Sciences**. v. 14, n. 4, p. 51-56, 2011.

ÁLVARES, C. A.; SVIDZINSKI, T.I.E.; CONSOLARO, M.E.L. Vulvovaginal candidiasis: host predisposing factors and yeast virulence. **J. Bras. Patol. Med. Lab.**, Rio de Janeiro, v. 43, n. 5, p. 319- 327, 2007.

ANDES, D.; NETT, J.; OSCHEL, P.; ALBRECHT, R.; MARCHILLO, K.; PITULA, A. Development and characterisation of an in vivo central venous catheter Candida albicans biofilm model. **Infect. Immun.** 72:6023-6031, 2004.

ANDRADE, Iara Pinheiro Barros. **Effects of vinegar on Candida Albicans after in vitro adherence to thermally activated acrylic resin.** 2006. 49 f. Dissertation (Master's Degree) - Department of Dentistry, University of Taubaté, Taubaté, 2006.

ANTUNES, R.M.P.; LIMA, E.O.; PEREIRA, M.S.V.; CAMARA, C.A.; ARRUDA, T.A.; CATÃO, R.M.R.; BARBOSA, T.P.; NUNES, X.P.; DIAS, C.S.; SILVA, T.M.S. In vitro antimicrobial activity and determination of the minimum inhibitory concentration (MIC) of phytoconstituents and synthetic products on bacteria and yeast-like fungi. **Rev Bras Farmacogn.** v. 16, n. 4, p. 517-524, 2006.

APEL, MA.; SOBRAL, M.; HENRIQUES, A.T. Composição química do óleo volatátil de Myrcianthes nativas da região sul do Brasil. **Rev Bras Farmacogn** 16: 402-407, 2006.

ARRUDA, T.A.; ANTUNES, R.M.P.; CATÃO, R.M.R.; LIMA, E.O.; SOUSA, D.P.; NUNES, X.P.; PEREIRA, M.S.V.; BARBOSA-FILHO, J.M.; CUNHA, E.V.L. Preliminary study of the antimicrobial activity of Mentha x villosa Hudson essential oil, rotundifolone and its analogues. **Rev Bras Farmacogn.** v. 16, p. 307-311, 2006.

ARWEILER, N.B.; DONOS, N.; NETUSCHIL, L.; REICH, E.; SCULEAN, A. Clinical and antibacterial effect of tea tree oil - a pilot study. **Clin Oral Investig.** v. 4, p. 70- 73, 2000.

ASEKUN, O.T.; GRIERSON, D.S.; AFOLAYAN, A.J. Effects of drying methods on the quality and quantity of the essential oil of Mentha longifolia L. subsp. capensis. **Food Chem** 101: 995-998, 2006.

AZEVEDO, N.F.; CERCA, F. Biofilms: in Health, in the Environment, in Industry. Porto: Publindustria, Produção de comunicação, Ltda, 2012.

AZEVEDO, N.R.; CAMPOS, I.F.P.; FERREIRA, H.D.; PORTES, T.A.; SANTOS, S.C.; SERAPHIN, J.C.; PAULA, J.R.; FERRI, P.H. Essential oil chemotypes in Hyptis suaveolens from Brazilian Cerrado. **Biochem Syst Ecol** 30: 205-216, 2002.

BAGGE, N.; HENTZER, M.; ANDERSEN, J.B.; CIOFU, O.; GIVSKOV, M.; H0IBY, N. Dynamics and spatial distribution of beta-lactamase expression in Pseudomonas aeruginosa biofilms. **Antimicrob Agents Chemother** 48: 1168-1174, 2004.

BAILLIE, G. S.; DOUGLAS, L. J. Role of dimorphism in the development of Candida albicans biofilms. **J. Med. Microbiol.** 48:671-679, 1999.

BARBEDO, L. S.; SGARBI, D. B. G. Candidiasis. **STD - J. Bras. Doenças Sex. Transm.**, Rio de Janeiro, v. 22, n. 1, p. 22-38, 2010.

BARBIERI, Dicler de SanfAnna Vitor. **Analysing the "in vitro" adherence of Streptococcus mutans and Candida albicans to the dental surface.** 2005. 110 f. Dissertation (Master's Degree in Microbiology) - Department of Basic Pathology, Biological Sciences Sector, Federal University of Paraná, Curitiba, 2005.

BASSOLE, I.H.N.; OUATTARA, A.S.; NEBIE, R.; OUATTARA, C.A.T.; KABORE, Z.I.; TRAORE, A.S. Chemical composition and antibacterial activities of the essential oils of

Lippia chevalieri and Lippia multifl ora from Burkina Faso. **Phytochemistry** 62: 209-212, 2003.

BATISTA, T.F.; RODRIGUES, M.C.S. Post-discharge surgical site infection surveillance in a teaching hospital in the Federal District, Brazil: a retrospective descriptive study from 2005-2010. **Epidemiol Serv Saúde**, Brasília. v. 21, n. 12, p. 253-64, 2012.

BENNETT, R. J.; UHL, A.M.; MILLER, G.M.; JOHNSON, D.A. Identification and characterisation of a Candida albicans mating pheromone. **Mol. Cell. Biol.** 23:8189- 8201, 2003.

BENKEBLIA, N. Antimicrobial activity of essential oil extracts of various onions (Allium cepa) and garlic (Allium sativum). **Lebensm-Wiss Technol**. v. 37, p. 263268, 2004.

BHAVANANI, S.M.; BALLOW, C.H. New agents for Gram-positive bacteria. **Curr Opin Microbiol**. v. 3 p. 528-534, 2000.

BIZZO, R.H.; HOVELL, C.M.A.; REZENDE, M.C. Essential oils in Brazil: general aspects, development and prospects. **Quim. Nova.** v. 32, n. 3, p. 588594,2009.

BRYANT, K.; MAXFIELD, C.; RALABAIS, G. Renal candidiasis in neonates with candiduria. **Paediatr Infect Dis J**; 18:959-63, 1999.

CALDERONE, R. A.; FONZIWA, W. A. Virulence factors of C. albicans. **Trends Microbiol.**, Cambridge, v. 9, p. 327-335. 2001.

CANILLAC, N.; MOUREY, A. Antibacterial activity of the essential oil of Picea excelsa on Listeria, Staphylococcus aureus and coliform bacteria. Food Microbiol 18:261-268, 2001.

CARVALHO-FILHO, J.L.S.; BLANK, A.F.; ALVES, P.B.; EHLERT, P.A.D.; MELO, A.S.;

CAVALCANTI, S.C.H.; ARRIGONI-BLANK, M.F.; SILVA-MANN, R. Influence of the harvesting time, temperature and drying period on basil (Ocimum basilicum L.) essential oil. **Rev Bras Farmacogn** 16: 24-30, 2006.

CASTRO, L.T.; COUTINHO, M.D.H.; GEDEON, C.C.; SANTOS, M.J.; SANTANA, J.W.; SOUZA, S.B.L. Mechanisms of resistance of Candida sp WWA to antifungal drugs. **Infarma**. v. 18, n. 9, 2006.

CASTRO, H. G. et al. Contribution to the study of medicinal plants: secondary metabolites. 2. ed. Viçosa: UFV, 2004a. 113 p.

CEGELSKI, L.; MARSHALL G. R.; G. R. ELDRIDGE.; HULTGREN, S. J. The biology and future prospects of antivirulence therapies. **Nature Rev. Microbiol**. v.6, n.1, p.17-27, 2008.

CHANDRA, J.; KUHN, D. M.; MUKHERJEE, P. K.; HOYER, L. L.; MCCORMICK, T.; GHANNOUM, M. A.. Biofilm Formation by the Fungal Pathogen Candida albicans: Development, Architecture, and Drug Resistance. **J. Bacteriol**. v.183, n.18, p. 5385- 5394, 2001.

CHENG, M.F.; YANG,Y.L.; YAO, T.J.; LIN, C.Y.; LIU, J.S.; TANG, R.B.; YU, K.W.; FAN, Y.H.; HSIEH, K.S.; HO, M.; LO, H.J. Risk factors for fatal candidemia caused by Candida albicans and non-albicans Candida species. **BMC Infectious Diseases**, v. 5, n.1, p.5, 2005.

CHEN, W.; VILJOEN, A. M. Geraniol - A review of a commercially important fragrance material. **South African Journal of Botany**, v. 76, n. 4, 2010.

CIMANGA, K.; KAMBU, K.; TONA, L.; APERS, S.; DE BRUYNE, T.; HERMANS, N.; TOTTÉ, J.; PIETERS, L.; VLIETINCK, A.J. Correlation between chemical composition and antibacterial activity of essential oils of some aromatic medicinal plants growing in the

Democratic Republic of Congo. **J Ethnopharmacol** 79: 213-220, 2002.

CLAFFEY, N. Essential oil mouthwashes: a key component in oral health management. **J Clin Periodontol**. v. 30, p. 22- 24, 2003.

COAD, B. R.; KIDD, S. E.; ELLIS, D. H.; GRIESSER, H. J. Biomaterials surfaces capable of resisting fungal attachment and biofilm formation. **Biotechnol. Adv.** v.32, n.2, p.296-307, 2014.

COLOMBO, A. L. et al. Epidemiology of candidemia in Brazil: a nationwide sentinel surveillance of candidemia in eleven medical centres. **J Clin Microbiol**. v. 44, n. 8, p. 2816-23, 2006.

COLOMBO, A.L. et al. High rate of non-albicans candidemia in Brazilian tertiary care hospitals. **Diagn Microbiol Infect Dis**, 34: 281-86, 1999.

COLOMBO, A. L.; GUIMARÃES, T. Epidemiologia das infecções hematogênicas por Candida spp. **Rev Soc Bras Med Trop**. v. 36. n. 5, p. 599-607, 2003.

CONNER, D.E. Naturally occurring compounds. In: DAVIDSON P.; BRANEN A.L. Antimicrobials in foods. **New York: Marcel Dekker**, Inc. 1993. p.441-68.

COSTA, P.D.; ANDRADE, N.J.; PASSOS, F.J.V.; BRANDÃO, S.C.C.; RODRIGUES, C.G.F. ATP-bioluminescence as a technique to evaluate the microbiological quality of water in food industry. **Braz Arch Biol Technol**. v. 47, n. 3, p. 399-405, 2013.

COUTO, R.C.; PEDROSA, T.M.G.; NOGUEIRA, J.M. Infecção Hospitalar - Epidemiologia, Controle e tratamento. 3ª ed. Rio de Janeiro, **Editora Médica e Científica**; 2003.

DELESPAUL, Q.; DE BILLERBECK, V.G.; ROQUES, C.G.; MICHEL, O. The antifungal activity of essential oils as determined by different screening methods. **J. Essent. Oil Res**. v. 12, p.256-266, 2000.

DE-SOUZA, M.M.; GARBELOTO, M.; DENEZ, K.; EGER-MANGRICH, I. Evaluation of the central effects of Bach florals in mice through specific pharmacological models. **Rev Bras Farmacogn** 16: 365-371, 2006.

DONLAN, R.M.; COSTERTON, J.W. Biofilms: survival mechanisms of clinically relevant microorganisms. **Clin Microbiol Rev.** v. 15, p.167-193, 2002.

DONLAN, R. M.. Biofilms: Microbial Life on Surfaces. **Emerg Infect Dis.** v.8, n.9, p.881-890, 2002.

DUARTE, M.C.T. et al. Activity of essential oils from Brazilian medicinal plants on Escherichia coli. **Journal of Ethno pharmacology**. v. 111, p. 197-201, 2007.

DUPONT, B. Clinical manifestations and management of candidosis in the compromised patient. In: Warnock DW, Richardson MD editors. Fungal infection in the compromised patient, 2nd ed. **New York: John Wiley & Sons**, 55-83, 1991.

EDWARDS, J.E.JR. Invasive Candida infections...Evolution of a fungal pathogen. **N Engl J Med**; 324:1060-2, 1991.

ESEN, S.; LEBLEBICIOGLU, H. Prevalence of nosocomial infections at intensive care units in Turkey: a multicentre 1-day point prevalence study. **Scand J Infect Dis.** 36: 144-8, 2004.

FINE, D.H.; FURGANG, D.; BARNETT, M.L.; DREW, C.; STEINBERG, L.; CHARLES, C.H.; VINCENT, J.W. Effect of an essential oil-containing antiseptic mouthrinse on plaque and salivary Streptococcus mutans levels. **J Clin Periodontol**. v. 27, p. 157-161, 2000.

FRANCO, J.; NAKASHIMA, T.; FRANCO, L.; BOLLER, C. Chemical composition and in vitro antimicrobial activity of the essential oil of Eucalyptus cinerea F. Mull. ex Benth., Myrtaceae, extracted at different time intervals. **Rev Bras Farmacogn** 15: 191-194, 2005.

GILBERT, P.; MCBAIN, A.J. & RICKARD, A.H. 2003. Formation of microbial biofilm in hygienic situations: a problem of control. **International Biodeterioration & Biodegradation.** v. 51, p. 245-248.

GIONGO, J.L.; VAUCHER, R.A.; FAUSTO, V.P.; QUATRIN, P.M.; LOPES, L.Q.S.; SANTOS, R.C.V.; GÚNDEL, A.; GOMES, *P;* STEPPE, M. Anti-Candida activity assessment of Pelargonium graveolens oil free and nanoemulsion in biofilm formation in hospital medical supplies. **Microbial Pathogeneses**. v. 100, p. 170-178, 2016.

GUDLAUGSSON, O, et al. Attributable Mortality of Nosocomial Candidemia, **Revisited. Clin Infec Dis**. v.37 p. 1172-77, 2003.

GUIMARÃES, M.M.Q.; ROCCO, J.R. Prevalence and prognosis of patients with ventilator-associated pneumonia in a university hospital. **Rev Bras Pneumol**. 22(4):339-46, 2006.

HALL-STOODLEY, L.; COSTERTON, W.J.; STOODLEY, P. Bacterial biofilms: from the natural environment to infectious diseases. **Nat. Rev. Microbiol.** 2:95-108, 2004.

HALL-STOODLEY, L.; STOODLEY, P. Biofilm formation and dispersal and the transmission of human pathogens. **Trends Microbiol** 1: 7-10, 2005.

HAMMER, K.A.; CARSON, C.F.; RILEY, T.V. Antimicrobial activity of essential oils and other plant extracts. **J Appl Microbiol.** 86: 985-990, 1999.

HEAD, K.A. Natural approaches to prevention and treatment of infections of the lower urinary tract. **Altern Med Rev.** 13: 227-44, 2008.

HOOD, J.R.; WILKINSON, J.M.; CAVANAGH, H.M.A. Evaluation of common antibacterial screening methods utilised in essential oil research. **J Essent Oil Res** 15: 428-433, 2003.

HOTA, B. Contamination, Disinfection, and Cross Colonisation: Are Hospital Surfaces Reservoirs for Nosocomial Infection? **Clin Infect Dis.** v. 39 p. 1182-89, 2004.

JANTAN, I.B.; MOHARAN, B.A.K.; SANTHANAM, J.; JAMAL, J.A. Correlation between chemical composition and antifungal activity of the essential oils of eight Cinnamomum species. **Pharm. Biol.**, 46(6): 405-12, 2008.

JARVIS, W.R. Epidemiology of nosocomial fungal infections, with emphasis on Candida species. **Clin Infect Dis.** v. 20, p. 1526-1530, 1995.

JIROVETZ, L. et al. Purity, antimicrobial activities and olfactoric evaluations of geraniol/nerol and various of their derivatives. **Journal of Essential Oil Research.** v. 19, n. 3, p. 288-91, 2007.

JURCISEK, J.A.; BAKALETZ, L.O. Biofilms formed by nontypeable Haemophilus influenzae in vivo contain both double-stranded DNA and type IV pilin protein. **J Bacteriol** 189: 3868-3875, 2007.

KALSI, J; ARYA, M; WILSON, P; MUNDY, A. Hospital-acquired urinary tract infection. **Int J Clin Pract.** v. 57, p. 388-91, 2003.

KELLY, SL et al . **Biochem Soc Trans**, 21: 1034-38, 1993.

KIPANGA, N.P.; LUYTEN, W. Influence of serum and polystyrene plate type on stability of Candida albicans biofilms. **Journal of Microbiological Methods**. v.139, p.8-11, 2017.

KHAN, M. S. A, et al. Virulence and Pathogenicity of Fungal Pathogens with Special Reference to Candida albicans. Combating Fungal Infections. In: AHMAD, I., ET AL. **Combating Fungal Infection**: problems and remedy. Berlin: Springer. p.21-45, 2010.

KHANUJA, S.P.S.; SHASANY, A.K.; PAWAR, A.; LAL, R.K.; DAROKAR, M.P.; NAQUI, A.A.; RAJKUMAR, S.; SUNDARESAN, V.; LAL, N.; KUMAR, S. Essential oil constituents and RAPD makers to establish species relationship in Cymbopogon Spreng. (Poaceae). **Biochemical Systematics and Ecology**. v. 33, p. 171-186, 2005.
KUNIN, C.M. Urinary tract infections: detection, prevention and management. 5 ed. Baltimore: Williams and Wilkins, 1997.

LACAZ, Carlos da Silva. Candidiasis. **EPU EDUSP**, São Paulo, p. 190, 1980.

LACERDA, R.A. **Hospital infection and its relationship with the evolution of health care practices**. In: Lacerda RA. Infection Control in Surgical Centres - Facts, Myths and Controversies. São Paulo (SP): Atheneu; p. 9-23, 2003.

LAMBERT, R.J.; SKANDAMIS, P.N.; COOTE, P.J.; NYCHAS, G.J. A study of the minimum inhibitory concentration and mode of action of oregano essential oil, thymol and carvacrol. **J Appl Microbiol** 91: 453-462, 2001.

LAWRENCE, J.R.; KORBER, D.R.; HOYLE, B.D.; COSTERTON, J.W. & CALDWELL, D.E. Optical sectioning of microbial biofilms. **Journal of Bacteriology**. v. 173, p. 6558-6567, 1991.

LEAL, T.C.A. de B.; FREITAS, S. de P.; SILVA, J.F. da; CARVALHO, A.J.C. de. Evaluation of the effect of seasonal variation and harvest time on the leaf essential oil content of lemon balm (Cymbopogon citratus (DC) Stapf). **Revista Ceres**. v.48, n. 278, p. 445-453, 2001.

LENZ, A.P.; WILLIAMSON, K.S.; PITTS, B.; STEWART, P.S.; FRANKLIN, M.J. Localised gene expression in Pseudomonas aeruginosa biofilms. **Appl Environ Microbiol** 74: 4463M471, 2008.

LIMA, I.O.; OLIVEIRA, R.A.G.; LIMA, E.O.; FARIAS, N.M.P.; SOUZA, E.L. Antifungal activity of essential oils on Candida species. **Rev Bras Farmacogn**. 16(2):197-201, 2006.

LIS-BACHIN, M.; DEANS, S.G. Bioactivity of selected plant essential oils against Listeria monocytogenes. **J Appl Bacteriol** 82: 759-762, 1997.

LOPES, H.V.; TAVARES, W. Projeto Diretrizes - Associação Médica Brasileira (AMB) e Conselho Federal de Medicina (CFM)**; Sociedade Brasileira de Infectologia e Sociedade Brasileira de Urologia**. Urinary Tract Infections: Diagnosis, 2004.

LOPES, J et al. Decrease in Candida albicans strains with reduced susceptibility to fluconazole following changes in prescribing policies. **J Hosp Infect**, 48:122-2, 2001.

LORENZI, H.; MATOS, F.J.A. Plantas medicinais no Brasil: nativas e exóticas. Instituto Plantarum de Estudos da Flora, Nova Odessa, São Paulo, 2002.

LUCCHETTI, G.; SILVA, J.A.; UEDA, Y.M.S.; PEREZ, D.C.M.; MIMICA, J.M.L. Urinary tract infections: analysis of the frequency and sensitivity profile of agents causing urinary tract infections in patients with chronic bladder catheterisation. **Bras Patol Med Lab**. v. 41, n. 6, p. 383-389, 2005.

MAGDALENA, Matta de Henning; PERRONE, Marianella. Factors determining pathogenicity in relation to the ecology of Candida albicans in the oral cavity. **Acta Odontol. Venez.**, Caracas, v. 39, n. 2, 2001.

MAI-PROCHNOW, A.; LUCAS-ELIO, P.; EGAN, S.; THOMAS, T.; WEBB, J.S.; SANCHEZ-AMAT, A.; KJELLEBERG, S. Hydrogen peroxide linked to lysine oxidase activity facilitates biofilm differentiation and dispersal in several gramnegative bacteria. **J Bacteriol** 190: 5493-5501, 2008.

MALLAVARAPU, G.R.; RAO, B.R.R.; KAUL, P.N.; RAMESH, S.; BHATTACHARYA, A.K. Volatile constituents of the essential oils of the seeds and the herb of palmarosa (Cymbopogon martinii (Roxb.) Wats. var. motia Burk.). **Flavour Fragrance J**. v.13, p.167-169, 1998.

MARTINS, C.A.P. et al. Presence of Candida spp in patients with chronic pyriodontitis. **Ciênc. Odontol. Bras**, São José dos Campos, v. 5, n.3, p. 75-85, 2002.

MARTINS, P. **Epidemiologia das Infecções em centro de terapia intensiva de adulto (thesis)**. Belo Horizonte (MG): University of Minas Gerais; 2006.

MASSON, P.; MATHESON, S.; WEBSTER, A.C.; CRAIGER, J.C. Metaanalyses in Prevention and Treatment of Urinary Tract Infections. **Infect Dis Clin North Am.** 23: 355-85, 2009.

MCDOUGALD, D. et al. Should we stay or should we go: mechanisms and ecological consequences for biofilm dispersal. **Nat Rev Microbiol.** v.10,p. 39-50, 2012.

MERMEL, L.A. Prevention of intravascular catheter-related infections. **Ann Intern Med**, v. 132, n. 5, p. 391-402, 2000.

MIMS, C.; PLAYFAIR, J.; ROITT, L.; WAKELIN, D.; WILLIAMS, R. **Urinary tract infections**. In: MIMS, C; PLAYFAIR, J; ROITT, L; WAKELIN, D; WILLIAM, S. R. Medical microbiology. São Paulo: Manole. p.221-8, 2000.

MINISTRY OF HEALTH (BR). Issues guidelines and norms for the prevention and control of hospital-acquired infections: Ordinance No. 2.616, of 12 May 1998. **Official Gazette**, Federative Republic of Brazil, Brasília (DF), Jul 1998.

MORSCHHÀUSER, J. The genetic basis of fluconazole resistance development in Candida albicans. **Biochem Biophys Acta**, 1587: 240-48, 2002.

MOURA, B.E.M.; CAMPELO, A.D.M.S.; BRITO, D.P.C.F.; BATISTA, A.M.O.; ARAÚJO, D.E.M.T.; OLIVEIRA, D.S.D.A. Hospital infection: prevalence study in a public teaching hospital. **Brazilian Journal of Nursing**. Brasília 2007 Jul-Aug; 60(4):416-21.

MUNOZ, P et al. Frequency and clinical significance of bloodstream infections caused by C. albicans strains with reduced susceptibility to fluconazole. **Diagn Microbiol Infect Dis**, 44: 163-67, 2002.

NASCIMENTO, C.F.P.; NASCIMENTO, C.A.; RODRIGUES, S.C.; ANTONIOLLI, R.A.; SANTOS, O.P.; JÚNIOR, B.M.A.; TRINDADE, C.R. Antimicrobial activity of essential oils: a multifactorial approach to methods. **Brazilian Journal of Pharmacology**. 17(1): 108-113, Jan./Mar. 2007.

NETO JR., R.N. Urologia prática. 4 ed. São Paulo: Atheneu, 1999.

NOBILE, J.C.; NETT, E.J.; ANDES, R.D.; MITCHELL P.A. Function of Candida albicans Adhesin Hwpl in Biofilm Formation. **Eukaryotic cell**, Oct. 2006, p. 16041610 Vol. 5, No. 10.

NOSTRO, A.; BLANCO, A.R.; CANNATELLI, M.A.; ENEA, V.; FLAMINI, G.; MORELLI, I.; ROCCARO, A.S.; ALONZO, V. Susceptibility of methicillin-resistant staphylococci to oregano essential oil, carvacrol and thymol. **FEMS Microbiol Lett** 230: 191-195, 2004.

NOVAIS, T.S.; COSTA, J.F.O.; DAVID, J.P.L.; DAVID, J.M.; QUEIROZ, L.P.; FRANÇA, F.; GIULIETTI, A.M.; SOARES, M.B.P.; SANTOS, R.R. Antibacterial activity in some plant extracts from the Brazilian semi-arid region. **Rev Bras Farmacogn** 13(Supl. 2): 5-8, 2003.

NUNES, X.P.; MAIA, G.L.A.; ALMEIDA, J.R.G.S.; PEREIRA, F.O.; LIMA, E.O. Antimicrobial activity of the essential oil of Sida cordifolia L. **Rev Bras Farmacogn**. v.16, p. 642-644, 2006.

NWAUGO, V. O.; ONYEAGBA, R. A.; UMEHAM, S. N.; AZU, N.. Effect Of Physicochemical Properties And Attachment Surfaces On Biofilms In Cassava Mill Effluent Polluted Oloshi River, Nigeria. **Estud. Biol**. v.29, n.66, p.53-61, 2007.

OLIVEIRA, F.P.; LIMA, E.O.; SIQUEIRA JÚNIOR, J.P.; SOUZA, E.L.; SANTOS, B.H.C.; BARRETO, H.M. Effectiveness of Lippia sidoides Cham. (Verbenaceae) essential oil in inhibiting the growth of Staphylococcus aureus strains isolated from clinical material. **Rev Bras Farmacogn**. v. 16, p. 510-516, 2006.

OLIVEIRA, R.A.G.; LIMA, E.O.; SOUZA, E.L.; VIEIRA, W.L.; FREIRE, K.R.L.; TRAJANO, V.N.; LIMA, I.O.; SILVA-FILHO, R.N. Interference of Plectranthus amboinicus (Lour.) Spreng essential oil on the anti-Candida activity of some clinically used antifungals. **Rev Bras Farmacogn**. v. 17, p. 186-190, 2007.

OLIVEIRA, R.A.G.; LIMA, E.O.; VIEIRA, W.L.; FREIRE, K.R.L.; TRAJANO, V.N.;

LIMA, I.O.; SOUZA, E.L.; TOLEDO, M.S.; SILVA-FILHO, R.N. Study of the interference of essential oils on the activity of some antibiotics used in the clinic. **Rev Bras Farmacogn** 16: 77-82, 2006a.

OLIVEIRA, D.R.D.R.; MAFFEI, C.M.L.; MARTINEZ, R. Hospital urinary infection by yeasts of the genus candida. **Rev Ass Med Brasil**; 47(3): 231-5, 2001.

OLIVEIRA, R.N.; DIAS, I.J.M.; CÂMARA, C.A.G. Comparative study of the essential oil of Eugenia punicifolia (HBK) DC. from different localities in Pernambuco. **Rev Bras Farmacogn** 15: 39-43, 2005.

OPALCHENOVA, G.; OBRESHKOVA, D. Comparative studies on the activy of basil - an essential oil from Ocimum basilicum L. - against multidrug resistant clinical isolates of the genera Staphylococcus, Enterococcus and Pseudomonas by using different test methods. **J Microbiol Methods** 54: 105-110, 2003.

PAN, P.; BARNETT, M.L.; COELHO, J.; BROGDON, C.; FINNEGAN, M.B. Determination of the in situ bactericidal activity of an essential oil mouthrinse using a vital stain method. **J Clin Periodontol.** v. 27, p. 256-261, 2000.

PATTNAIK, S. et al. Antibacterial and antifungal activity of aromatic constituents of essential oils. **Microbes**, v. 89, n. 358, p. 39-46, 1997.

PEARSON, M.M.; LAURENCE, C.A.; GUINN, S.E.; HANSEN, E.J. Biofilm formation by Moraxella catarrhalis in vitro: roles of the UspA1 adhesin and the Hag haemagglutinin. **Infect Immun** 74: 1588-1596, 2006.

PERCIVAL et al. A review of the scientific evidence for biofilms in wounds. **Wound Repair Regen.** n. 20, p. 647-657, 2012.

PLOWMAN, R; GRAVES, N; ESQUIVEL, J; ROBERTS, J.A. An economic model to assess the cost and benefits of the routine use of silver alloy coated urinary catheters to reduce the risk of urinary tract infections in catheterised patients. **J Hosp Infect**. v. 48, p. 33-42, 2001.

POTZERNHEIM, M.C.L.; BIZZO, H.R.; VIEIRA, R.F. Analysis of the essential oils of three species of Piper collected in the region of the Federal District (Cerrado) and comparison with oils of plants from the region of Paraty, RJ (Atlantic Forest). **Rev Bras Farmacogn** 16: 246-251, 2006.

POZZATTI, P. In vitro activity of essential oils extracted from plants used as aspices against fluconazoleresistent and fluconazole-susceptible Candida spp. Can. **J. Microbiol.** 54(6): 950-6, 2008.

PRADE, S.S. Estudo Brasileiro da Magnitude das Infecões Hospitalares em Hospitais Terciários. **Rev Controle Infecção Hosp.** 1995;2(2).

PRASHAR, A.; HILI, P.; VENESS, G.R.; EVANS, S.C. Antimicrobial action of palmarosa oil (Cymbopogon martinii) on Saccharomyces cerevisiae. **Phytochemistry**, v. 63, n. 5, 2003.

PUREVDORJ-GAGE, B.; COSTERTON, W.J.; STOODLEY, P. Phenotypic differentiation and seeding dispersal in nonmucoid and mucoid Pseudomonas aeruginosa biofilms. **Microbiology** 151: 1569-1576, 2005.

RAO, E.V.S.P.; RAO, R.S.G.; PUTTANNA, K. Studies on in situ soil moisture conservation and additions of phosphorus and potassium in rainfed palmarosa (Cymbopogon martinii var. motia) in a semi-arid tropical region of India. **European Journal of Agronomy**, v. 14, p. 167-172, 2001.

RAO, R.R.B.; KAUL, N.P.; SYAMASUNDAR, V.K.; RAMESH, S. Chemical profiles of primary and secondary essential oils of palmarosa (Cymbopogon martini (Roxb.) Wats var.

motia Burk. **Industrial Crops and Products**. v. 21, p. 121-127, 2005.

RASOOLI, I.; MIRMOSTAFA, S.A. Antibacterial properties of Thymus pubescens and Thymus serpyllum essential oil. **Phytotherapy** 73: 244-250, 2002.

REHDER, V.L.G.; MACHADO, A.L.M.; DELARMELINA, C.; SARTORATTO, A.; FIGUEIRA, G.M.; DUARTE, M.C.T. Chemical composition and antimicrobial activity of Origanum applii and Origanum vulgare essential oils. **Rev Bras Pl Med**. v. 6, p. 67-71, 2004.

RIBEIRO, Evandro Leão. **Candida yeasts isolated from the mouth of children with Down's Syndrome: pheno-genotypic aspects, intrafamilial relationship and immunoglobulin profile**. 2008. 129 f Thesis (Doctorate) - Faculty of Health Sciences, University of Brasília, Brasília, 2008.

RIBEIRO, E. L., et al. Oral Candida albicans from children with Down Syndrome: Germ tube behaviour, exoenzymes and sensitivity to killer toxins. **Rev. Odonto Ciênc.**, Porto Alegre, v. 22, n. 57, 2007.

RIBEIRO, Mariceli Araujo. **Exoenzymes and molecular mechanisms of fluconazole resistance of C. albicans isolated from HIV-positive women**. 2002. 156 f. Thesis (Doctorate) - Institute of Biomedical Sciences, University of São Paulo, São Paulo, 2002.

SCHERMA, A. P. et al. Presence of Candida spp in the oral cavity of infants during the first four months of life. **Cienc. Odontol. Bras.**, São José dos Campos, v.7, n. 3, p. 79-86, 2004.

SEFI DKON, F.; ABBASI, K.; JAMZAD, Z.; AHMADI, S. The effect of distillation methods and stage of plant growth on the essential oil content and comoposition of Satureja rechingeri Jamzad. **Food Chem** 100: 1054-1058, 2007.

SEYMOUR, R. Additional properties and uses of essential oils. **J Clin Periodontol**. v. 30, p.

19-21, 2003.

SHAFI, P.M.; ROSAMMA, M.K.; JAMIL, K.; REDDY, P.S. Antibacterial activity of Syzygium cumini and Syzygium travancoricum leaf essential oil. **Fitoterapia**. 73: 414-416, 2002.

SHARMA, Y.; KHAN, A.L.; MANZOOR, N. Anti-Candida activity of geraniol involves disruption of cell membrane integrity and function. **Journal de Mycologie Médicale**. v. 26, p. 244-254, 2016.

SHERER, R.; WAGNER, R.; DUARTE, M.C.T.; GODOY, H.T. Composition and antioxidant and antimicrobial activities of clove, citronella and palmarosa essential oils. **Rev. Bras. Pl. Med., Botucatu**. v. 11, n. 4, p. 442-449, 2009.

SILVA, V.V.; DÍAZ, M.C.; FEBRÉ, N. Vigilancia de la resistencia de leveduras a antifúngicos. **Rev Chil infect**, 19 :56-65, 2002.

SIMÕES, M. Antimicrobial Strategies Effective Against Infectious Bacterial Biofilms. **Current Medicinal Chemistry**. v.18, n.14, p. 2129-2145, 2011.

SIMÕES, C.M.O.; SCHENKEL, E.P.; GOSMANN, G.; MELLO, J.C.P.; MENTZ, L.A.; PETROVICK, P.R. Farmacognosia: da planta ao medicamento. 3.ed. Editora da Universidade UFRGS / Editora da UFSC. Porto Alegre/Florianópolis, 2001.

SINGH, S.; SHARMA, P.; SHREEHARI, A. K. Dental Plaque Biofilm: An Invisible Terror in the Oral Cavity. **In The Battle Against Microbial Pathogens: Basic Science, Technological Advances and Educational Programmes** (pp. 422-428). Formatex, 2015.

SIQUEIRA, C.S.M.; BRITO, R.D.; SILVA, C.O.F. The use of Thyme Essential Oil (Thymus vulgaris) as a phytotherapeutic resource for acne vulgaris. **Revista Científica da FHO**

UNIARARAS. v. 3, n. 1, 2015.

SIQUI, A.C.; SAMPAIO, A.L.F.; SOUSA, M.C.; HENRIQUES, M.G.M.O.; RAMOS, M.F.S. Essential oils - anti-inflammatory potential. **Biotecnologia, Ciência e Desenvolvimento**. v. 16, p. 38-43, 2000.

STAMM, W.E. Catheter-associated urinary tract infections: epidemiology, pathogenesis and prevention. **Am J Med**, v. 91, Suppl 3B, p. 65S-71S, 1991.

STOODLEY, P.; SAUER, K.; DAVIES, D.G.; COSTERTON, J.W. Biofilms as complex differentiated communities. **Annu Rev Microbiol** 56: 187-209, 2002.

SUZUKI, Luis Claudio. **Development of biofilm formed by Candida albicans in vitro to study photodynamic therapy**. 2009. 48f. Thesis (Master of Science in Nuclear Technology - Materials)- Nuclear Energy Research Institute, University of São Paulo, São Paulo, 2009.

TAKAISI-KIKUNI, N.B.; TSHILANDA, D.; BABADY, B. Antibacterial activity of the essential oil of Cymbopogon densifl orus. **Phytotherapy** 71: 69-71, 2000.

TAMURA, K.N.; NEGRI, N.F.M.; BONASSOLI, A.L.; SVIDZINSKI, E.I.T. Virulence factors of Candida spp isolated from venous catheters and hands of hospital staff. **Revista da Sociedade Brasileira de Medicina Tropical**. v. 40, n. 1, p. 91-93, 2007.

TELCI, I.; BAYRAM, E.; YILMAZ, G.; AVCI, B. Variability in essential oil composition of Turkish basils (Ocimun basilicum L.). **Biochem Syst Ecol**. 34: 489497, 2006.

URIZAR, J.M. A. Candidíasis orales. **Rev. Iberoam. Micol**. Barcelona, v.19, p. 1721, 2002.

VALLE, G. C.; RENDE, J. C.; OKURA, M. H. Study of the Incidence of the Candida Genus in a Public University Hospital. **NewsLab**, São Paulo, v.17, n.101, p. 202-222, 2010.

VAN ZYL, R.L. et al. The biological activities of 20 nature identical essential oil constituents. **Journal of Essential Oil Research**, v.18, p.129-33, 2006.

VARGHESE, N.; YANG, S.; SEJWAL, P.; LUK, Y.Y. Surface control of blastospore attachment and ligand-mediated hyphae adhesion of Candida albicans. **Chem. Commun.** v.49, p.10418, 2013

VASUDEVAN, R. Biofilms: Microbial Cities of Scientific Significance. **Journal of Microbiology & Experimentation**, 1(3), 1-16, 2014.

VIDOTTO, V. et al. Adherence of Candida albicans and Candida du-bliniensis to buccal and vaginal cells. **Rev. Iberoam. Micol.**, Barcelona, v.20, p. 52-54, 2003.

VIEIRA, J. D. G., et al,. Candida albicans isolated from the oral cavity of children with Down syndrome: occurrence and growth inhibition by Streptomyces sp. **Rev. Soc. Bras. Med. Trop.**, Brasilia, v. 38, n. 5, p. 383-386, Sep/Oct 2005.

VILJOEN, A.M.; SUBRAMONEY, S.; VUUREN, S.F.V.; BASER, K.H.C.; DEMIRCI, B. The composition geografi cal variation and antimicrobial activity of Lippia javanica (Verbenaceae) leaf essential oils. **J Ethnopharmacol** 96: 271-277, 2005.

VUONG, C., et al. A crucial role for exopolysaccharide modification in bacterial biofilm formation, immune evasion, and virulence. **J Biol Chem**. v. 279 p. 5488154886, 2004a.

VUONG, C.; VOYICH, J.M.; FISCHER, E.R.; BRAUGHTON, K.R.; WHITNEY, A.R.; DELEO, F.R.; OTTO, M. Polysaccharide intercellular adhesin (PIA) protects Staphylococcus epidermidis against major components of the human innate immune system. **Cell Microbiol** 6: 269-275, 2004.

WEBB, J. S.; VAN DER MEI, H. C.; NIXON, M.; I. EASTWOOD, M.; GREENHALGH, M.; READ, S. J.; ROBSON, G. D.; HANDLEY, P. S. Plasticisers Increase Adhesion of the Deteriogenic Fungus Aureobasidium pullulans to Polyvinyl Chloride. **Appl Environ Microbiol**. v.65, n.8, p.3575-3581, 1999.

WINGETER, M. A.; GUILHERMETTI, E.; SHINOBU, C. S.; TAKAKI, I.; SVIDZINSKI,T. I. E. Microbiological identification and in vitro sensitivity of

Candida isolated from the oral cavity of HIV-positive individuals. **Revista da Sociedade Brasileira de Medicina Tropical**. v. 40, n.3, p.272-276, 2007.

WONG, E.S.; HOOTON, T.M. Guideline for prevention of catheterassociated urinary tract infections Centre for Diseases Control and Epidemiology. **Infect Control**. 2: 125-30, 1981.

ZARDO, V.; MEZZARI, A. Antifungals in Candida sp. infections. **News Lab** Ed.63, 2004.

ZHANG, L.; MAH, T.F. Involvement of a novel efflux system in biofilm-specific resistance to antibiotics. **J Bacteriol** 190: 4447-4452, 2008.

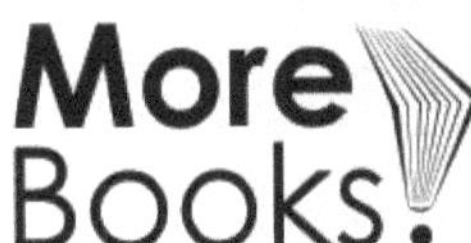

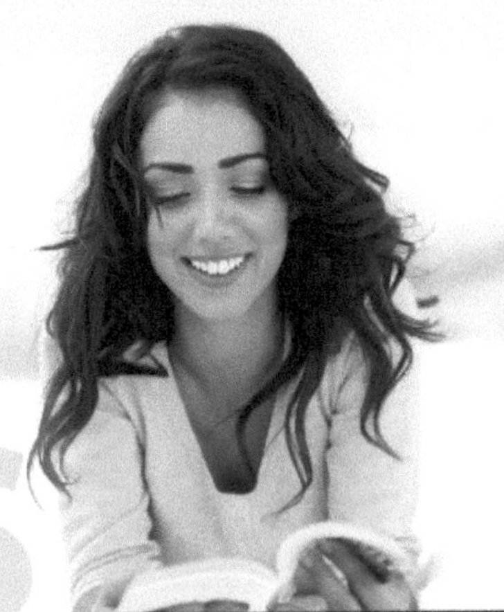

yes

I want morebooks!

Buy your books fast and straightforward online - at one of world's fastest growing online book stores! Environmentally sound due to Print-on-Demand technologies.

Buy your books online at
www.morebooks.shop

Kaufen Sie Ihre Bücher schnell und unkompliziert online – auf einer der am schnellsten wachsenden Buchhandelsplattformen weltweit! Dank Print-On-Demand umwelt- und ressourcenschonend produzi ert.

Bücher schneller online kaufen
www.morebooks.shop

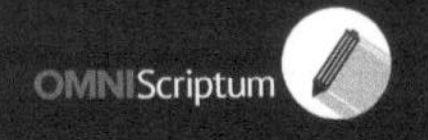

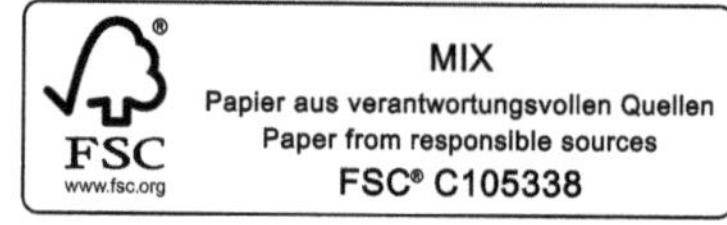

Printed by Books on Demand GmbH, Norderstedt / Germany